Coco's Magic

— Coco's Magic —

Written by **Jeongmin Ko K.M.D.** and
Hyojung Kwon K.M.D.
Illustrated by **Ji Eun Jeon**

Coco's Magic -Coco's Magic-

All That Korean Medicine

5th floor, Gosan-ro 4an-gil, Suseong-gu, Daegu, Republic of Korea

82-53-792-1565

www.allthatkm.com

Editor Project Bin

Designer Project Bin

ISBN 979-11-957979-1-2

   979-11-957979-0-5 (SET)

First Edition, March 2017

Coco's Magic

– Coco's Magic –

Character

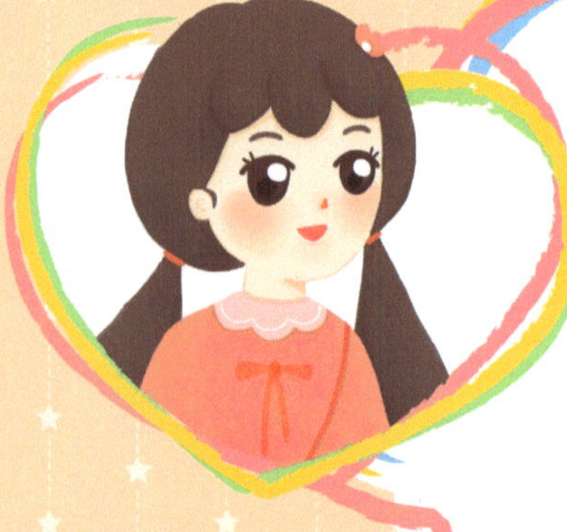

Coco

Coco is a lovely six-year-old girl who willingly helps friends in need. Her caring personality comes from the caring of her mother and grandmother.

Coco's Mom

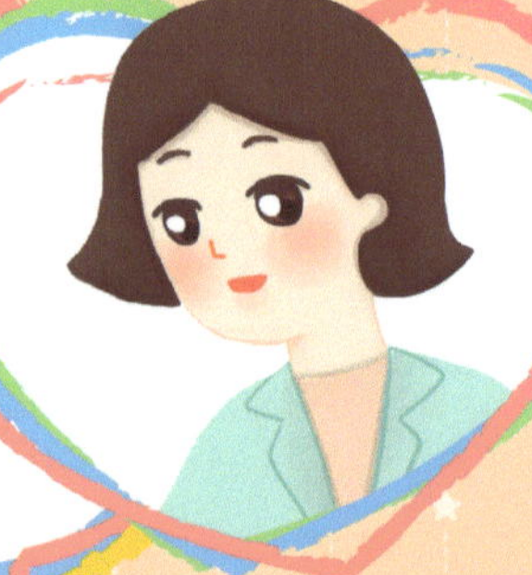

Coco's Mom is a Korean medical doctor who prescribes herbal medicine and treats with acupuncture, moxa, and cupping.

Mary

Mary is a shy girl who wants Coco to be her best friend. After getting over her shyness, she is all the more bright and active in the class!

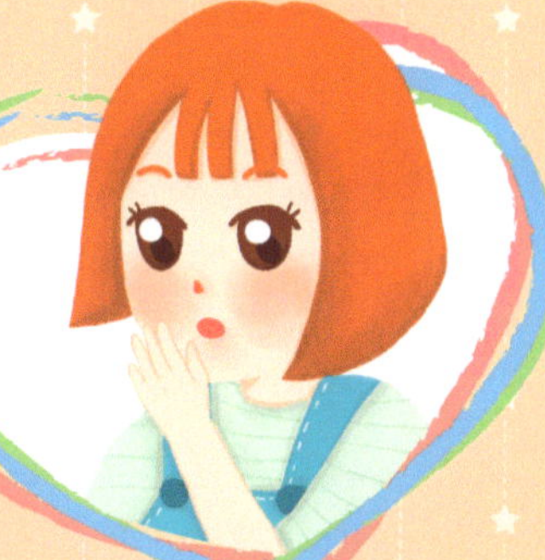

Tim

Tim is a bright boy, until he had bad dreams at nights and his brother kept waking him up. Little sleep makes Tim tired all the time.

Alice

Alice was born in her mother's country and moved to Korea when she turned six. She needs help with Korean language and table manners.

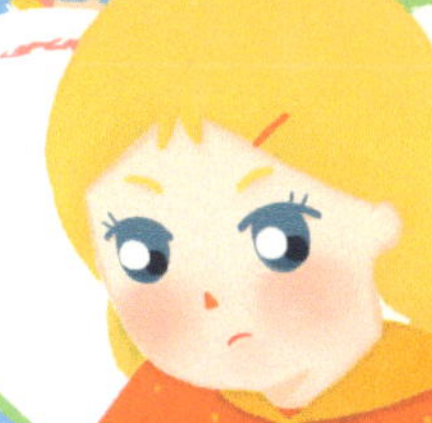

Justin

Every boy wants to be good at sports as Justin! Although bright and fast, one thing Justin is afraid of is insects!

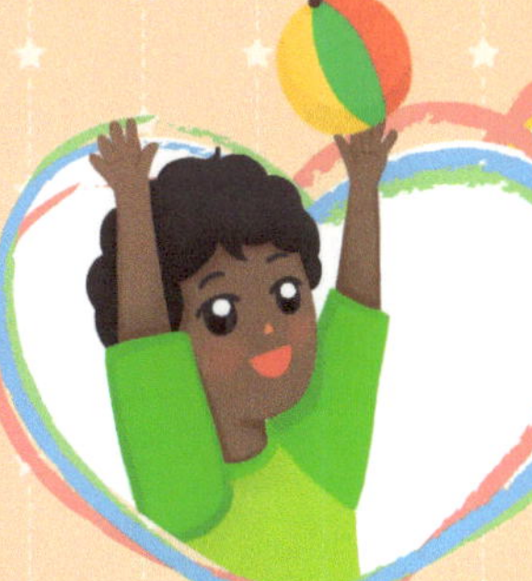

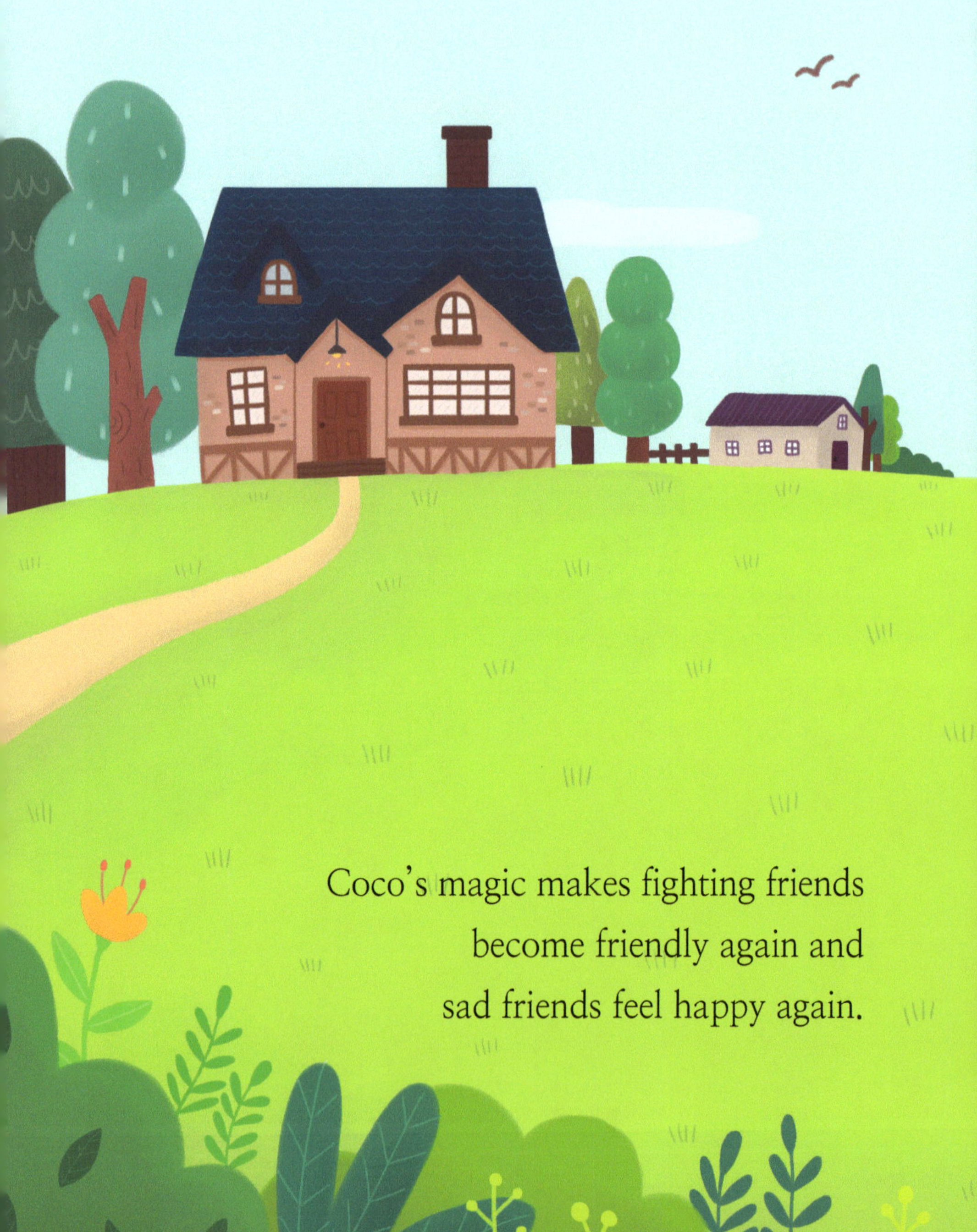

Coco is a six-year-old girl,
who has the magic of helping others.

Coco's magic makes fighting friends
become friendly again and
sad friends feel happy again.

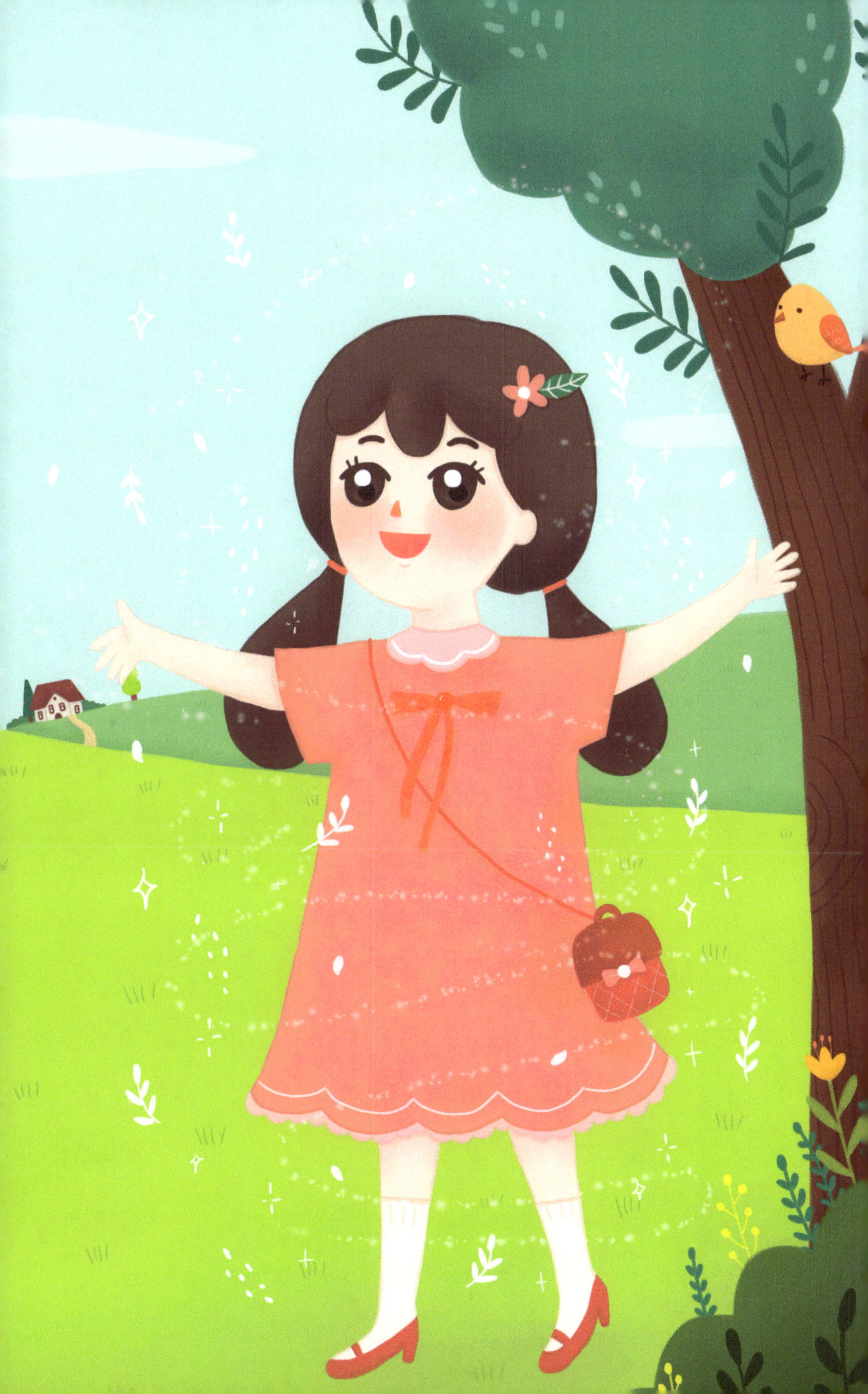

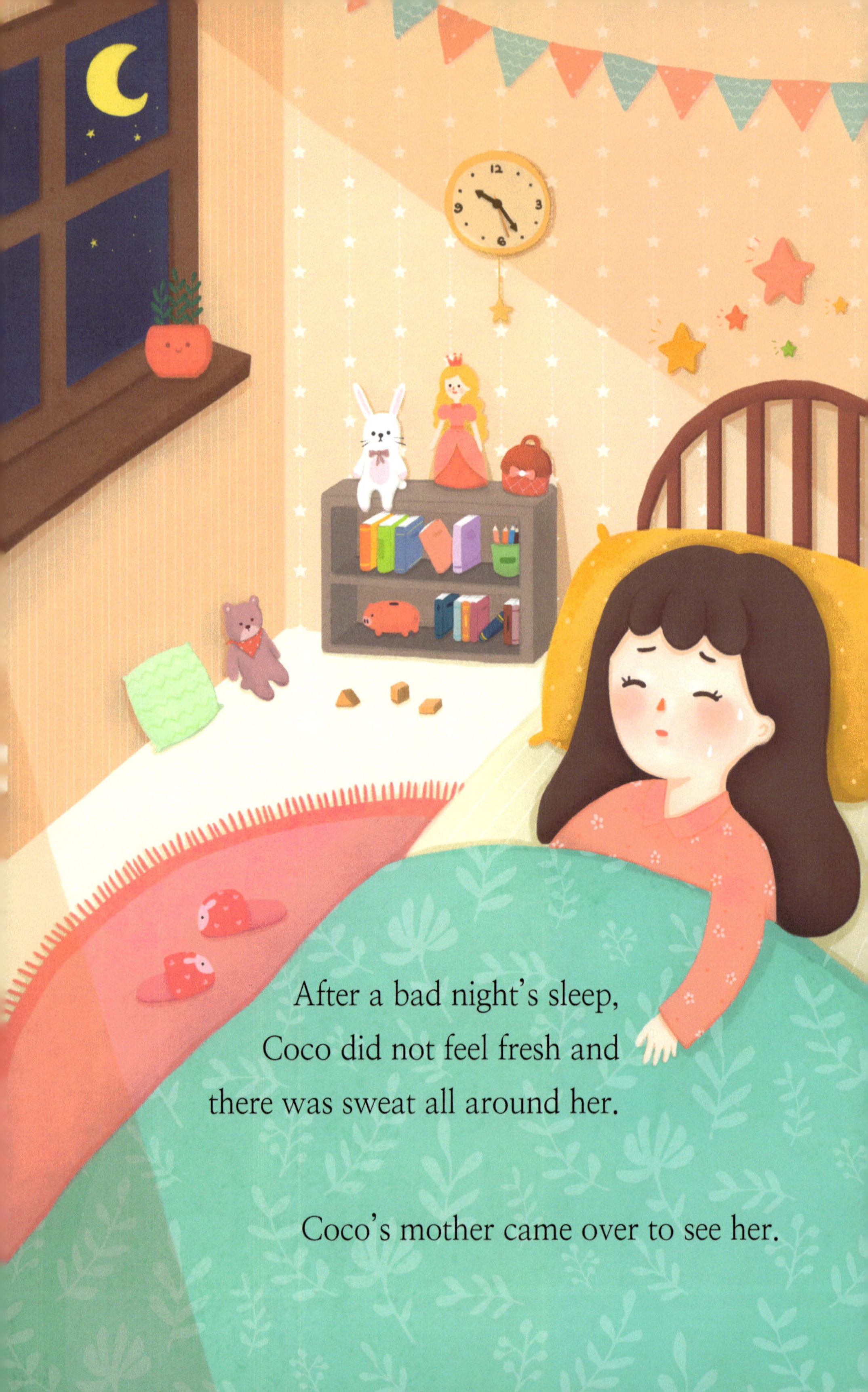

After a bad night's sleep,
Coco did not feel fresh and
there was sweat all around her.

Coco's mother came over to see her.

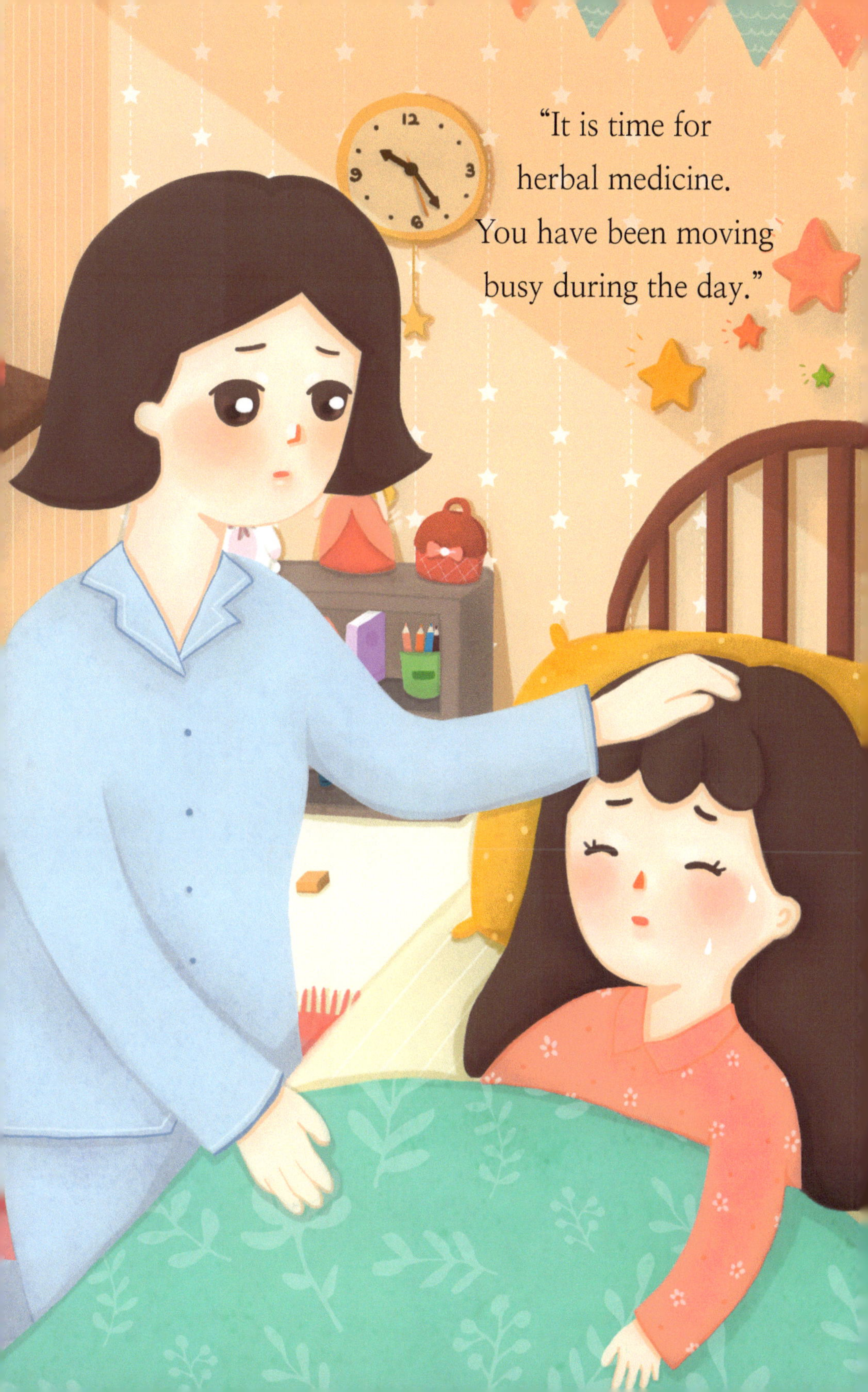
"It is time for
herbal medicine.
You have been moving
busy during the day."

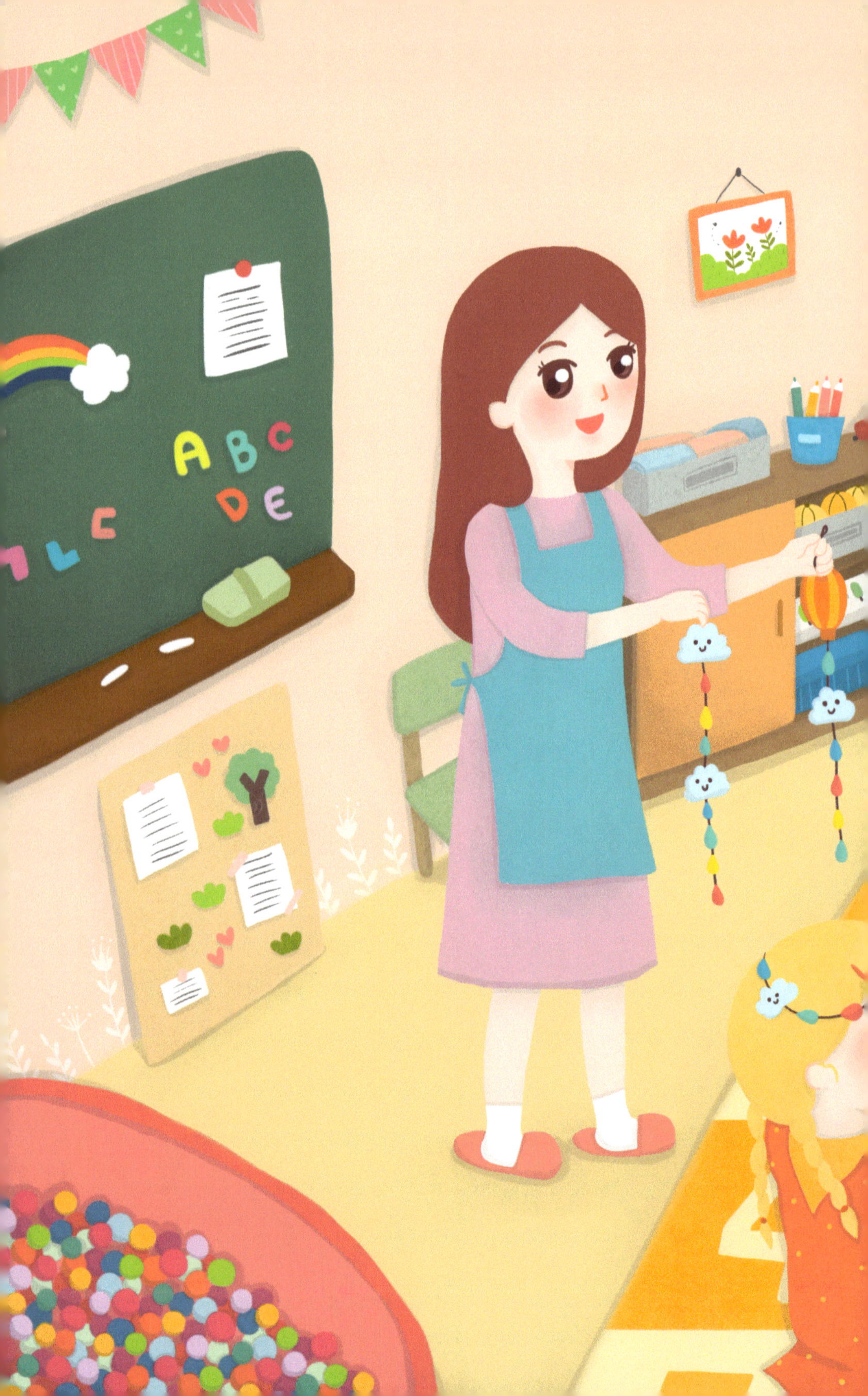

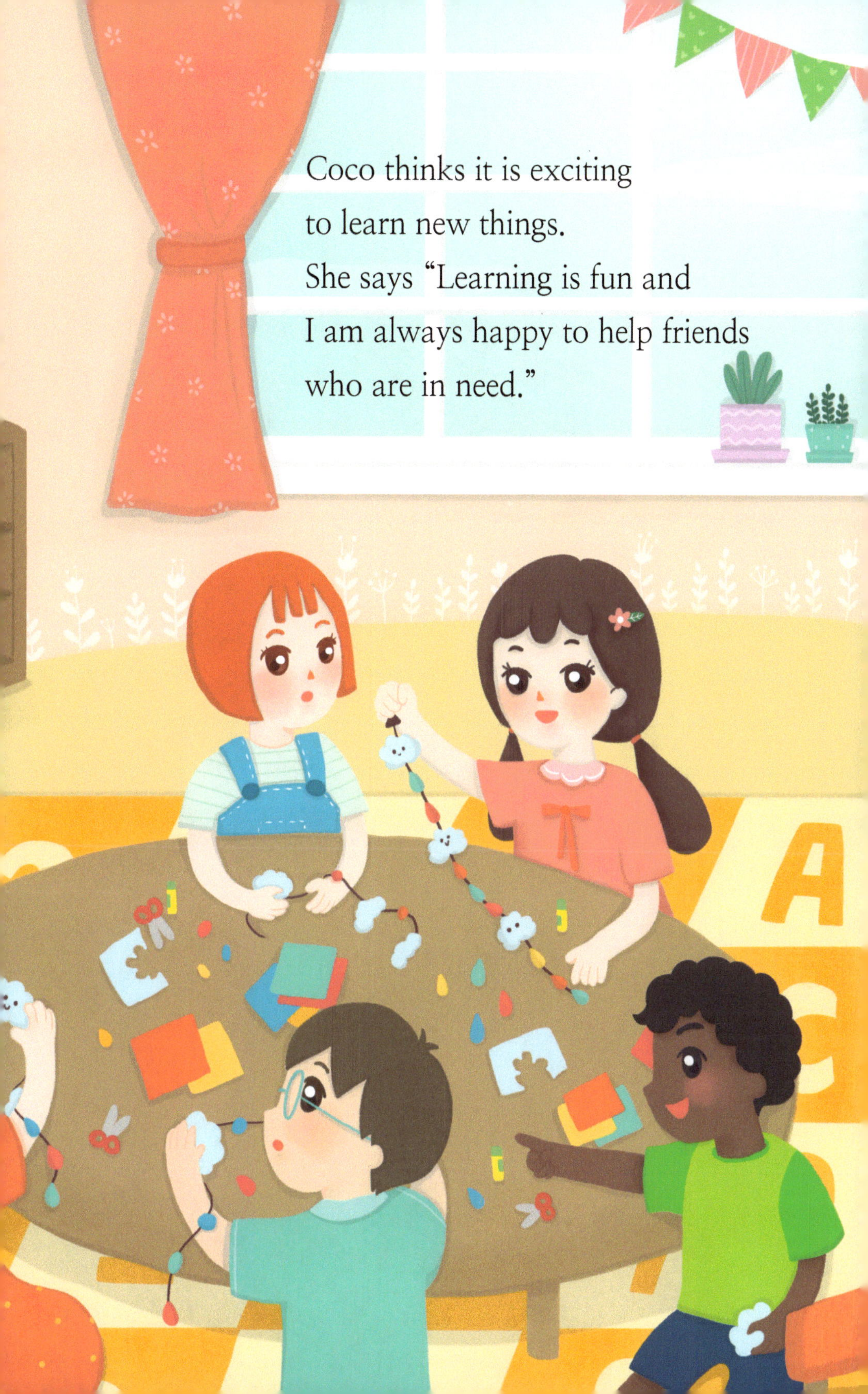

Coco thinks it is exciting
to learn new things.
She says "Learning is fun and
I am always happy to help friends
who are in need."

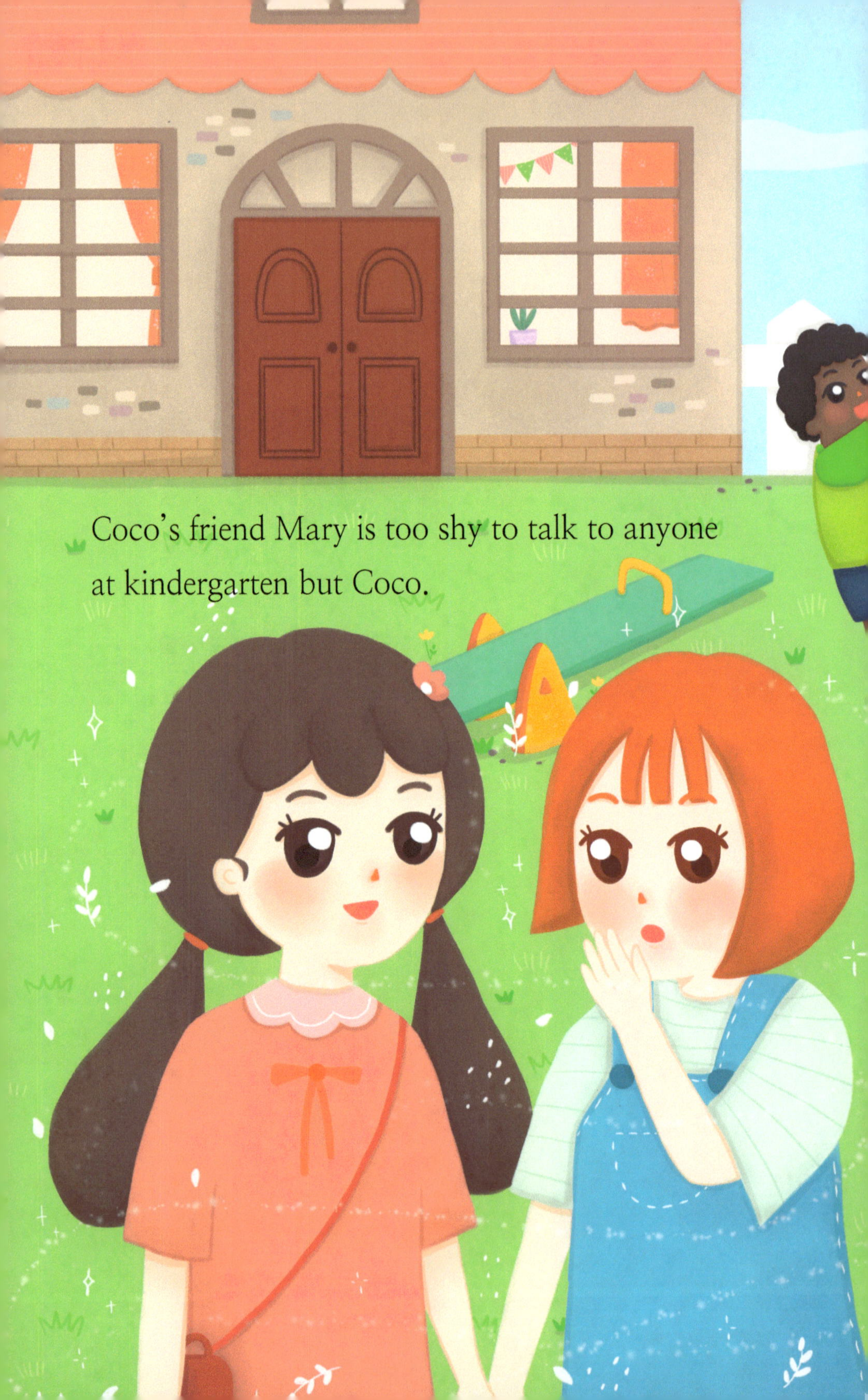

Coco's friend Mary is too shy to talk to anyone at kindergarten but Coco.

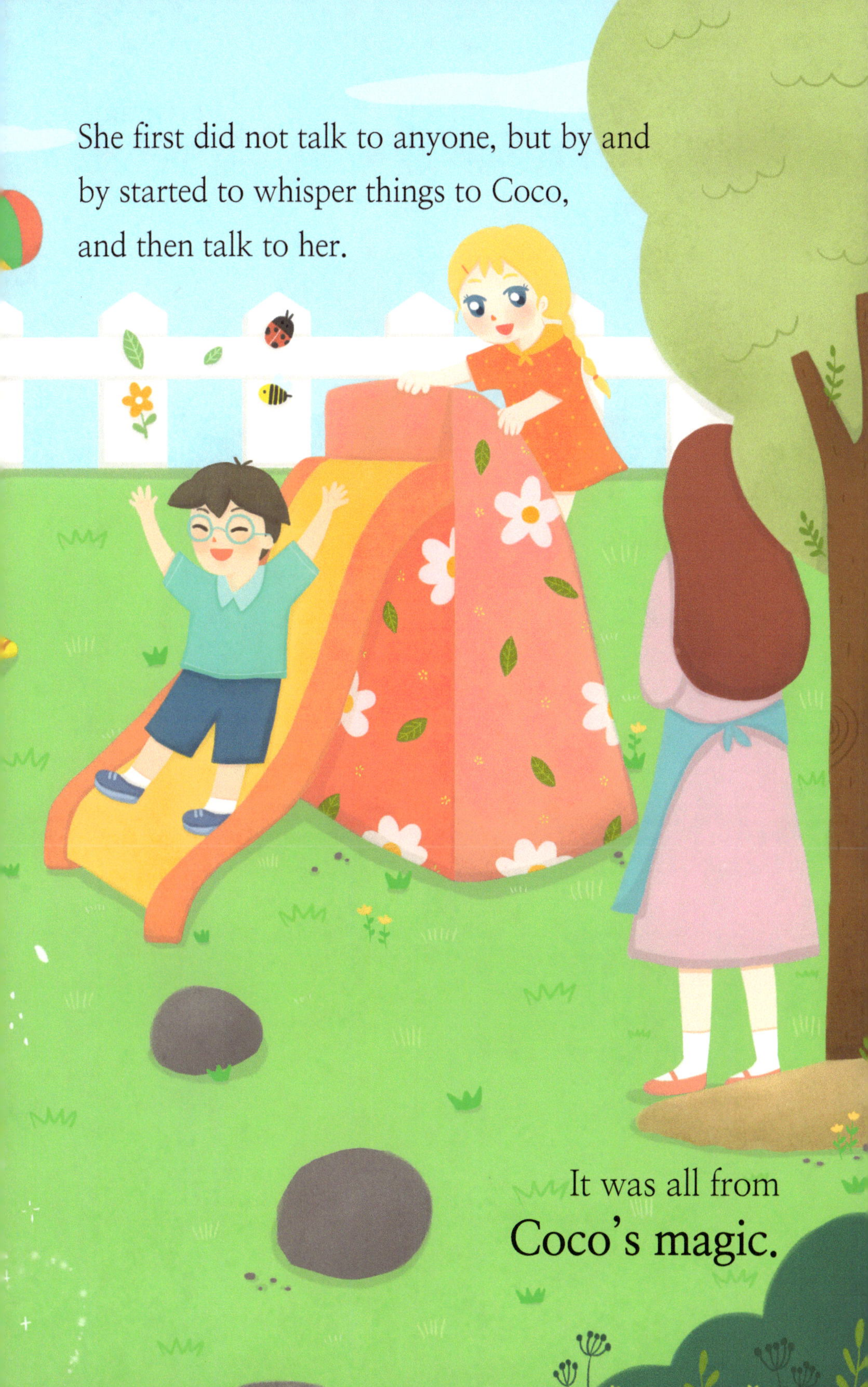

She first did not talk to anyone, but by and
by started to whisper things to Coco,
and then talk to her.

It was all from
Coco's magic.

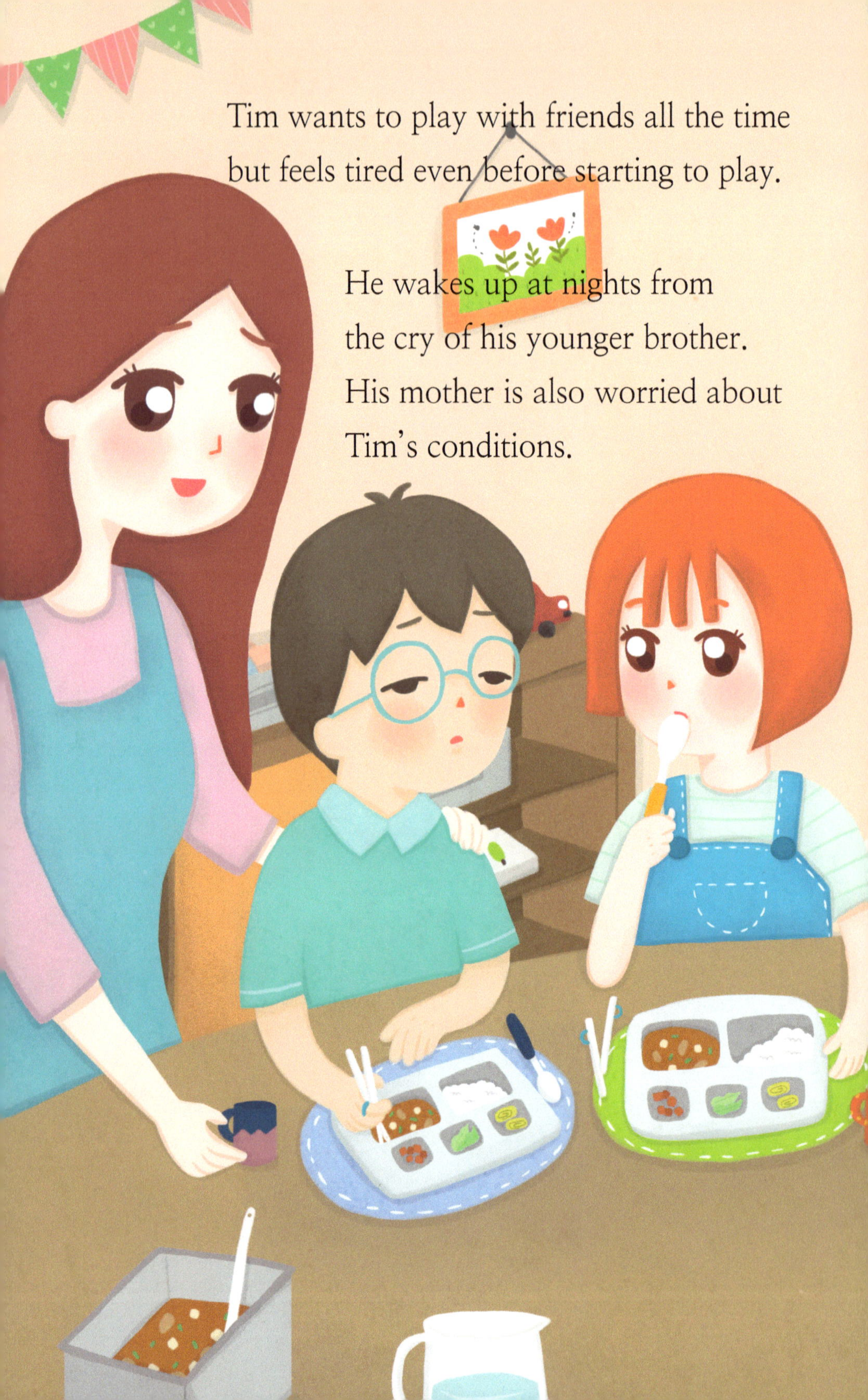

Tim wants to play with friends all the time
but feels tired even before starting to play.

He wakes up at nights from
the cry of his younger brother.
His mother is also worried about
Tim's conditions.

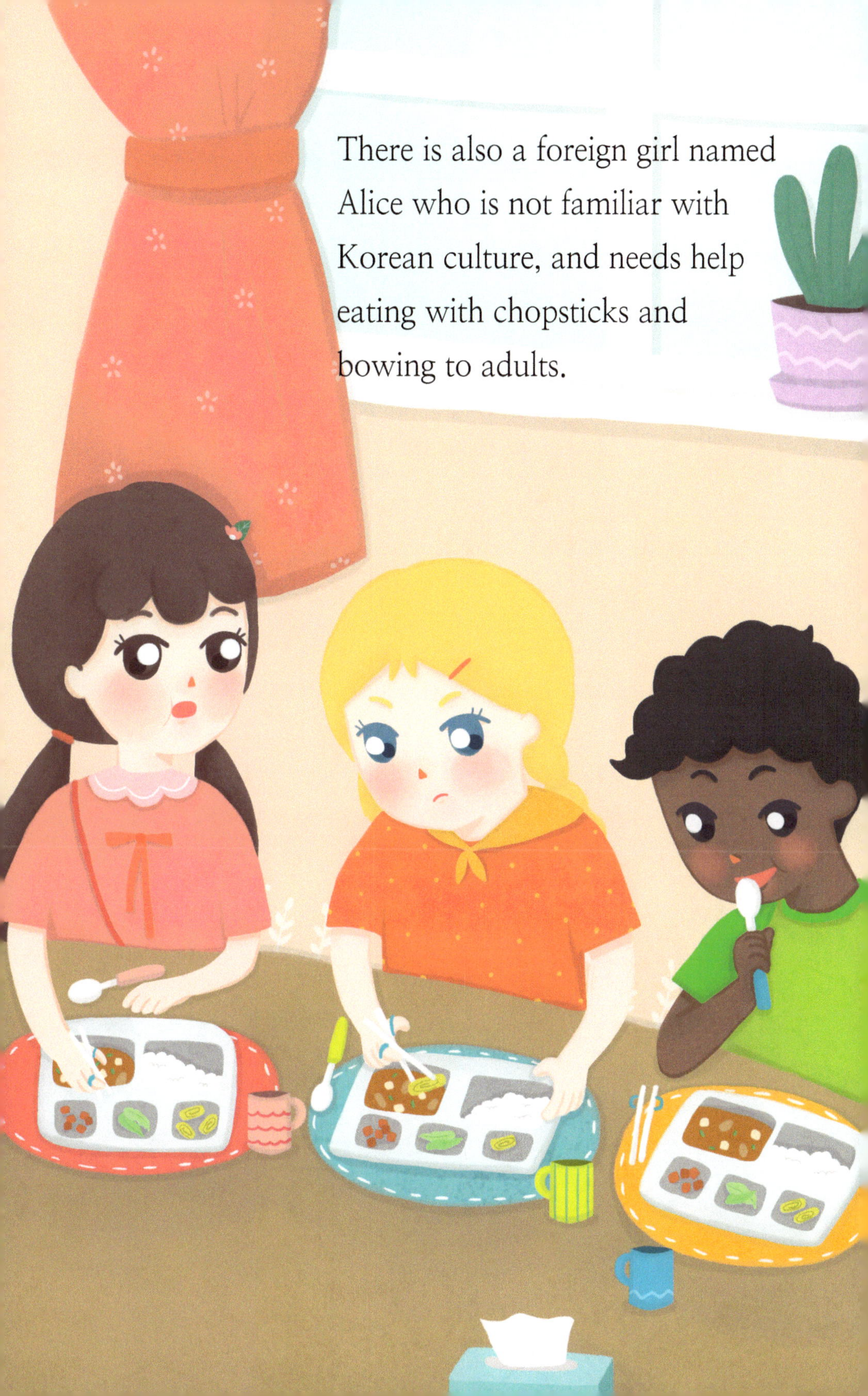

There is also a foreign girl named Alice who is not familiar with Korean culture, and needs help eating with chopsticks and bowing to adults.

Everybody at kindergarten loves Coco
because she has the magic of helping
those who are in need.

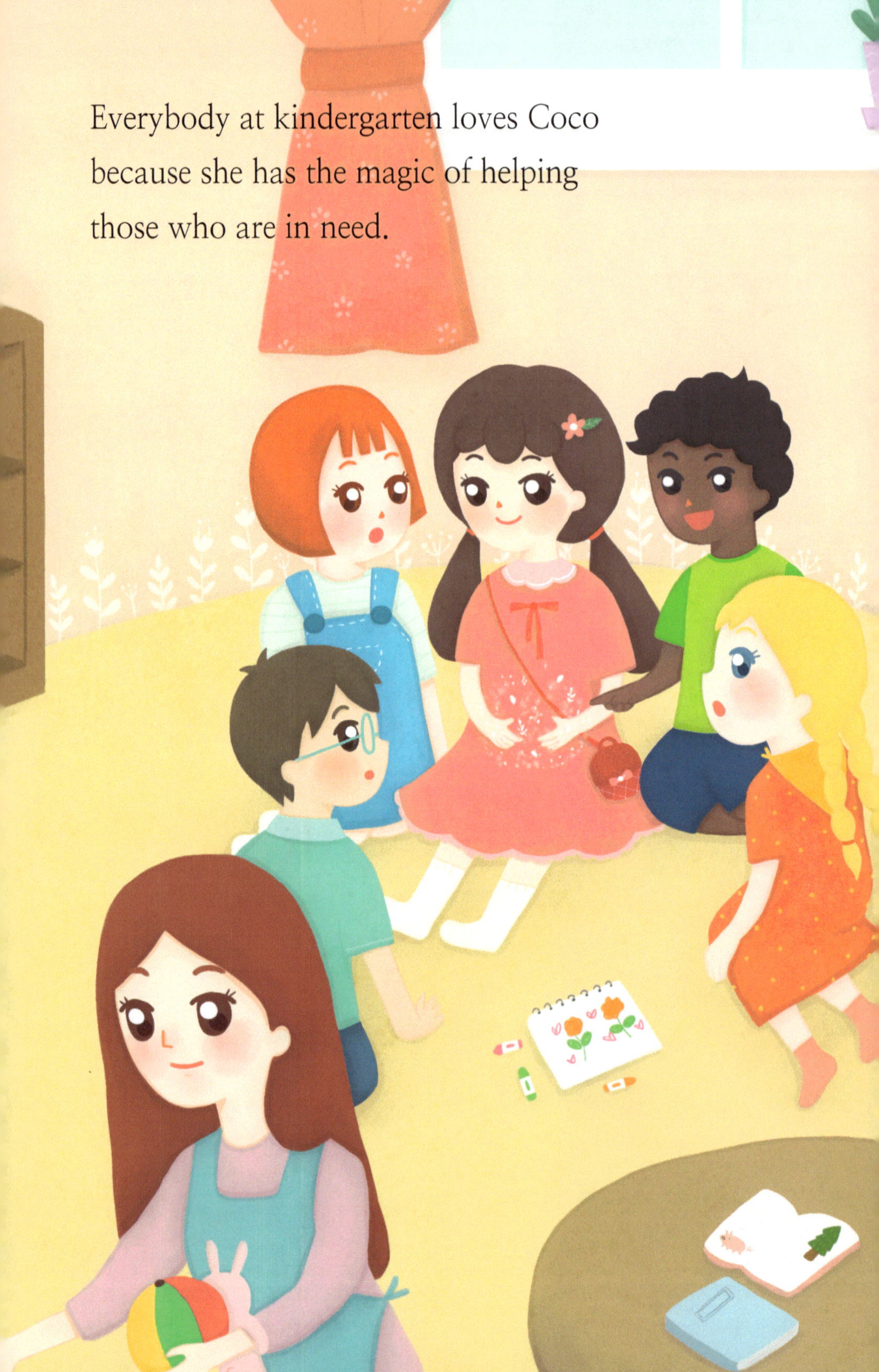

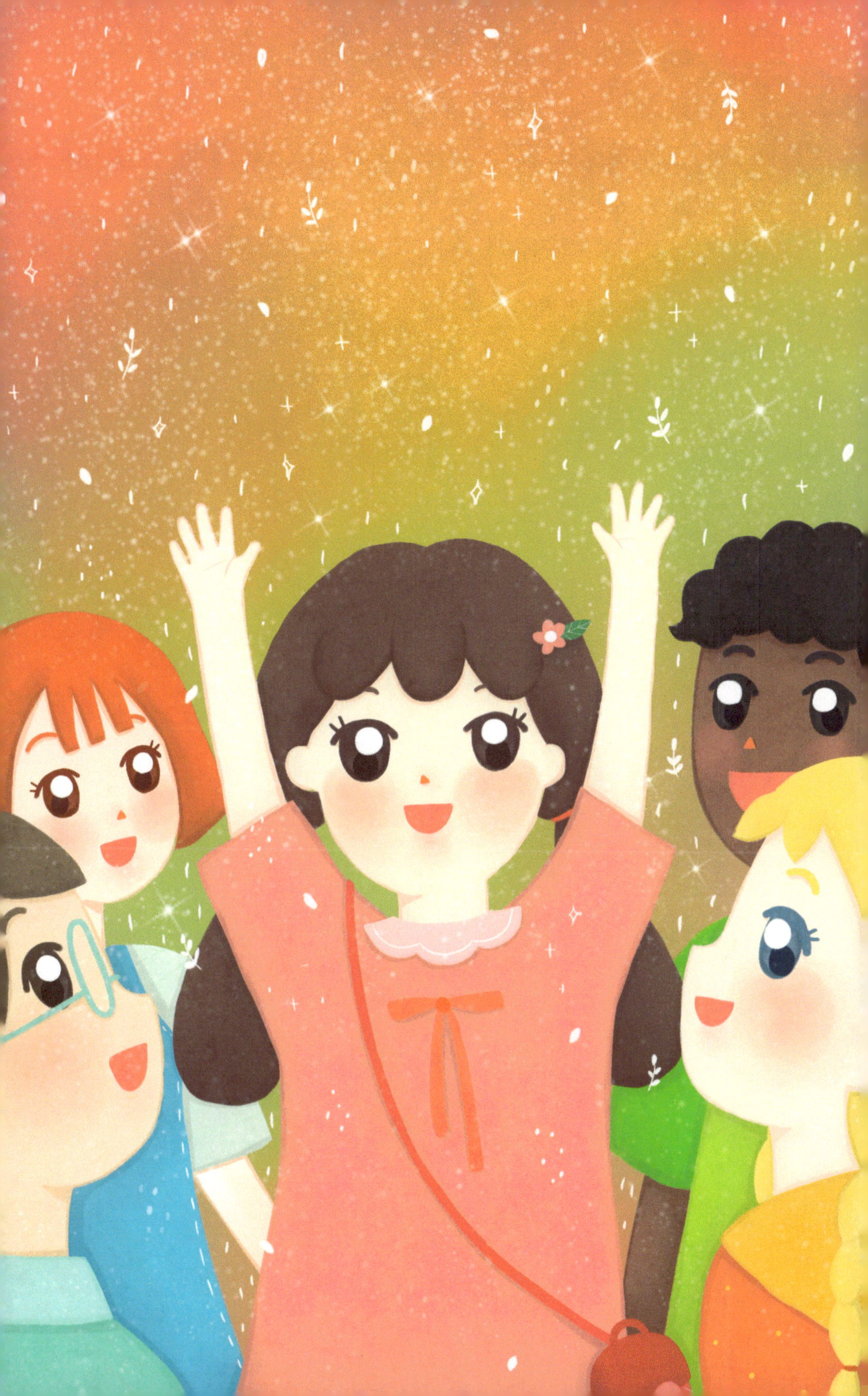

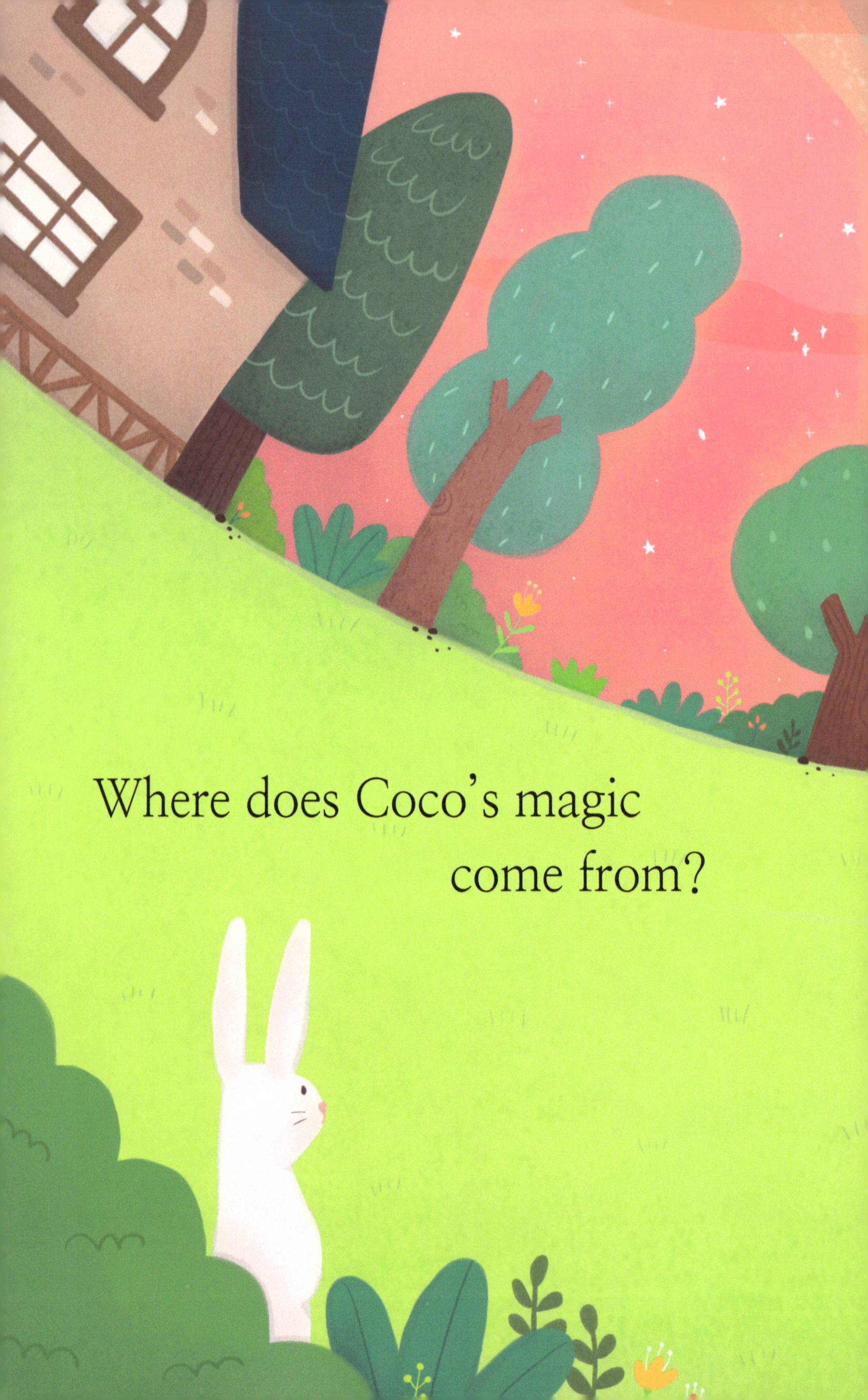

Where does Coco's magic
come from?

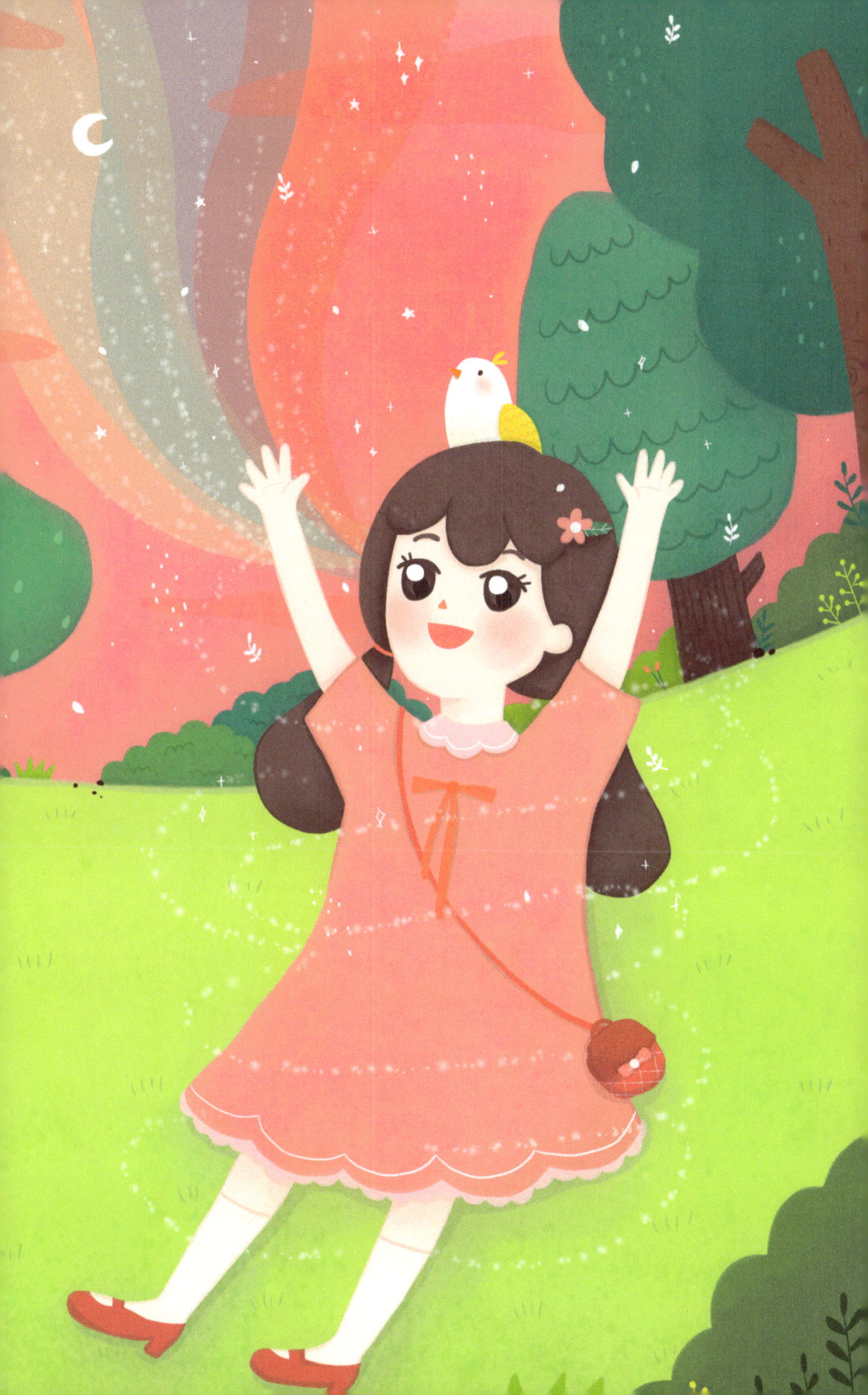

Her mother is a Korean medical doctor who treats patients with acupuncture and herbal medicine.
Coco takes herbal medicine frequently.
She even takes it when she is not sick.
Mostly it is in liquid form, and it is about one cup's amount at a time.

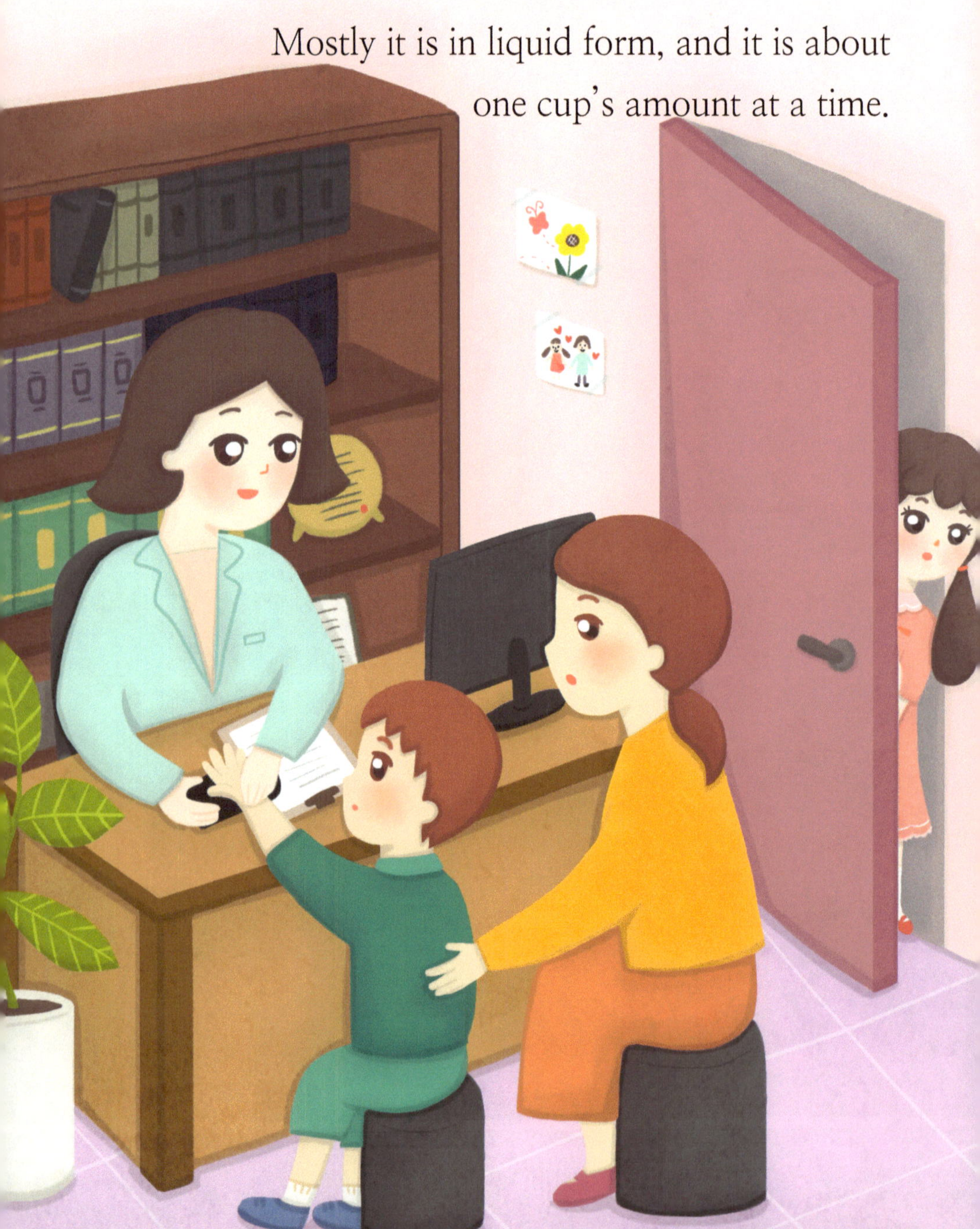

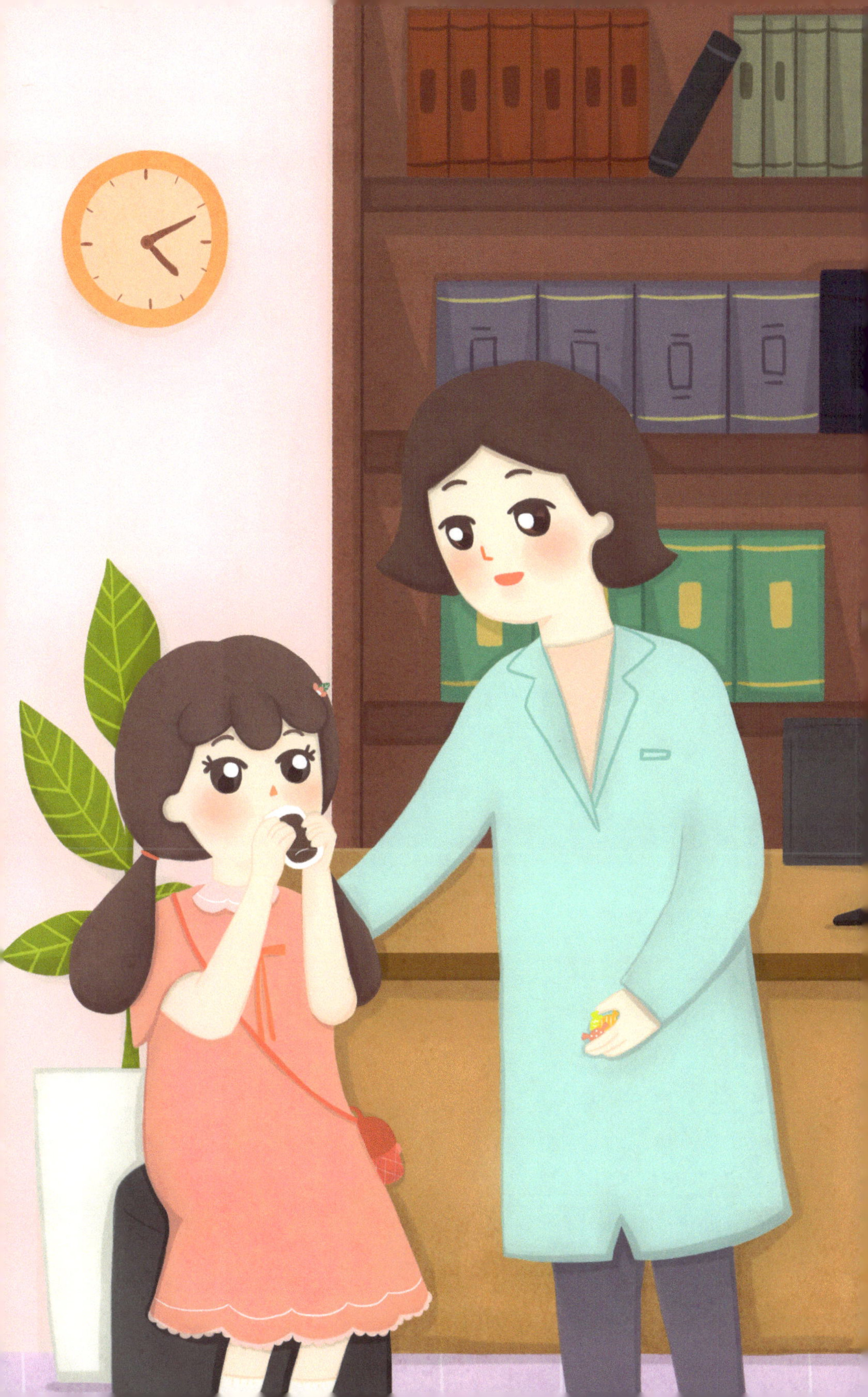

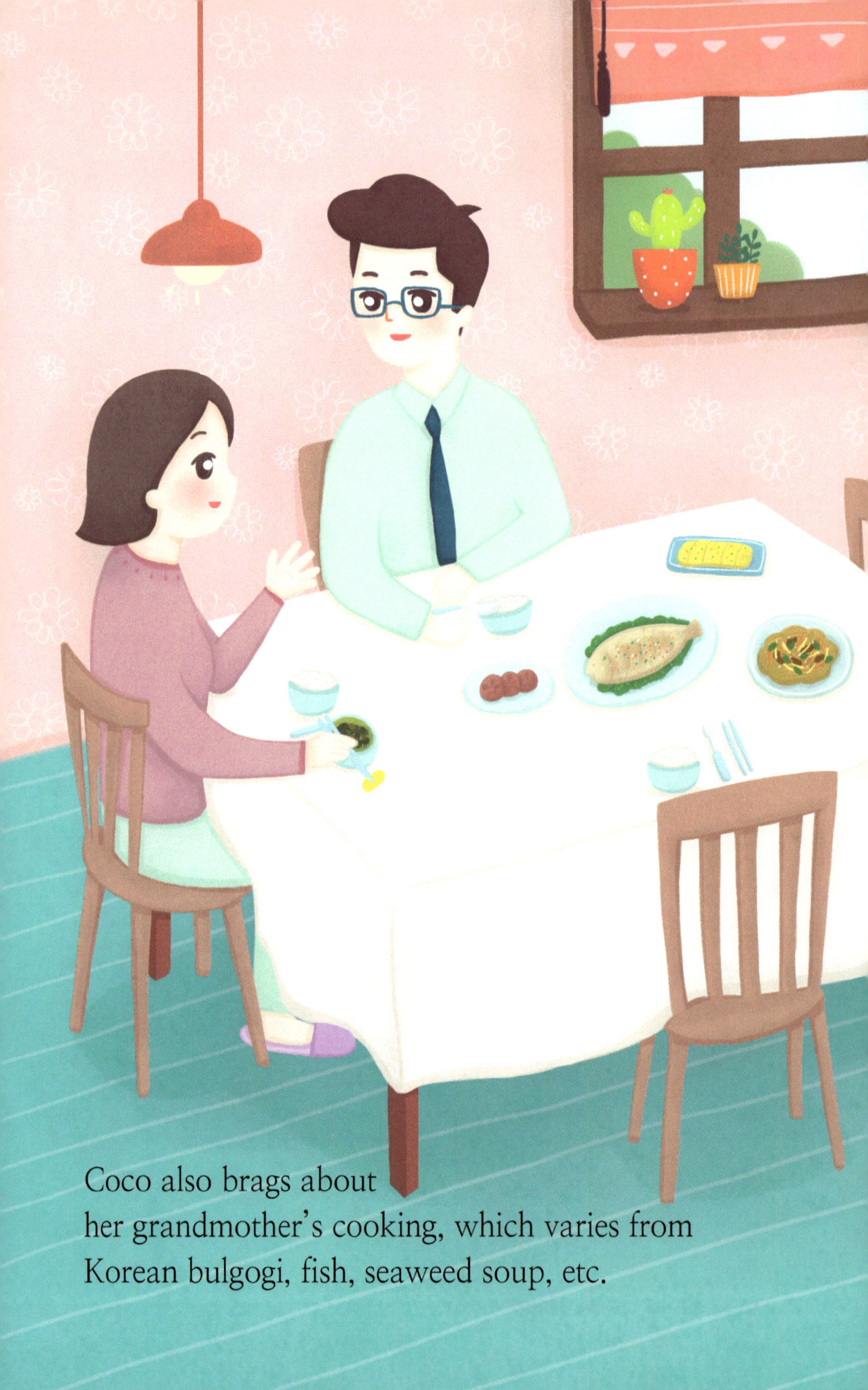

Coco also brags about
her grandmother's cooking, which varies from
Korean bulgogi, fish, seaweed soup, etc.

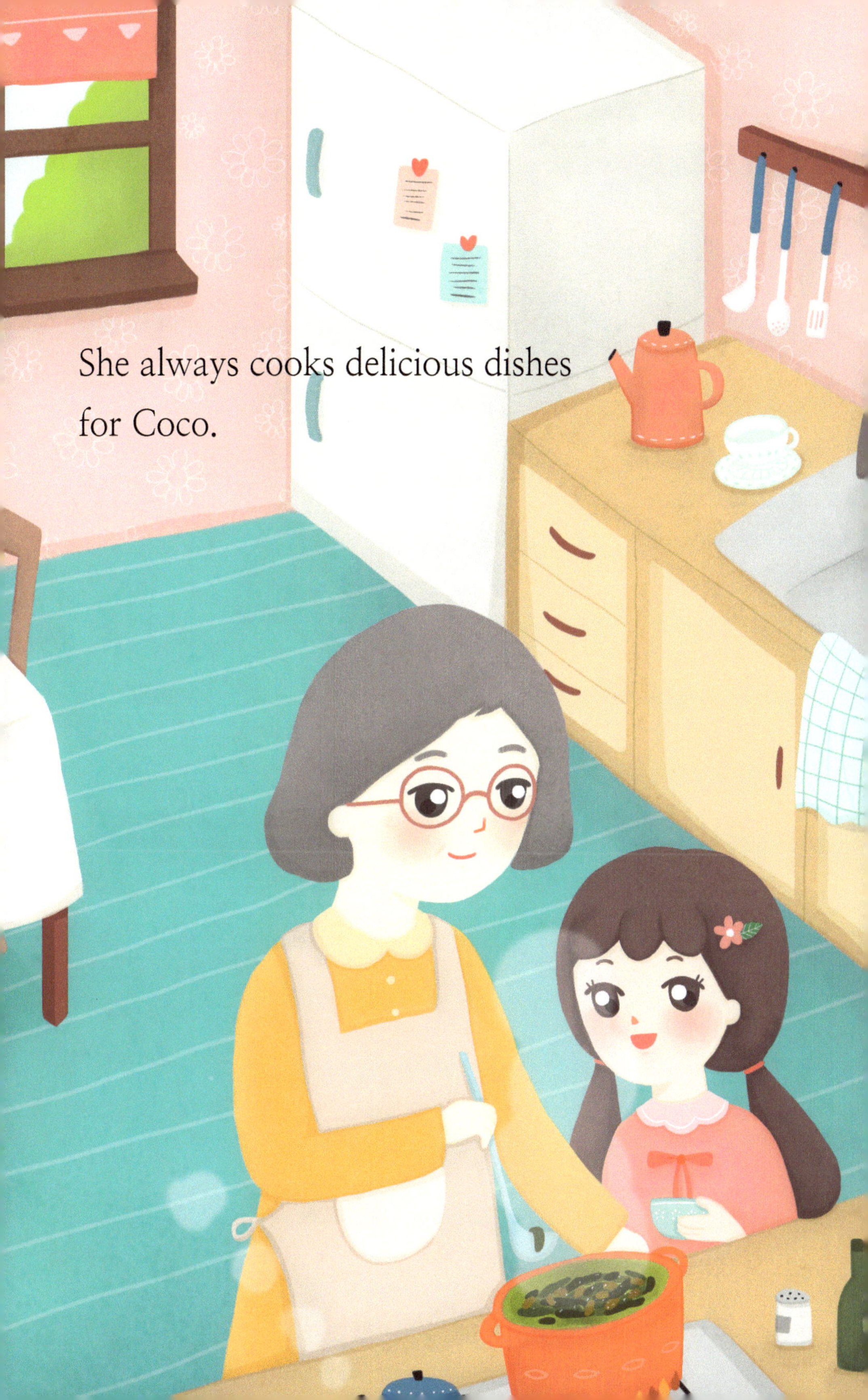
She always cooks delicious dishes
for Coco.

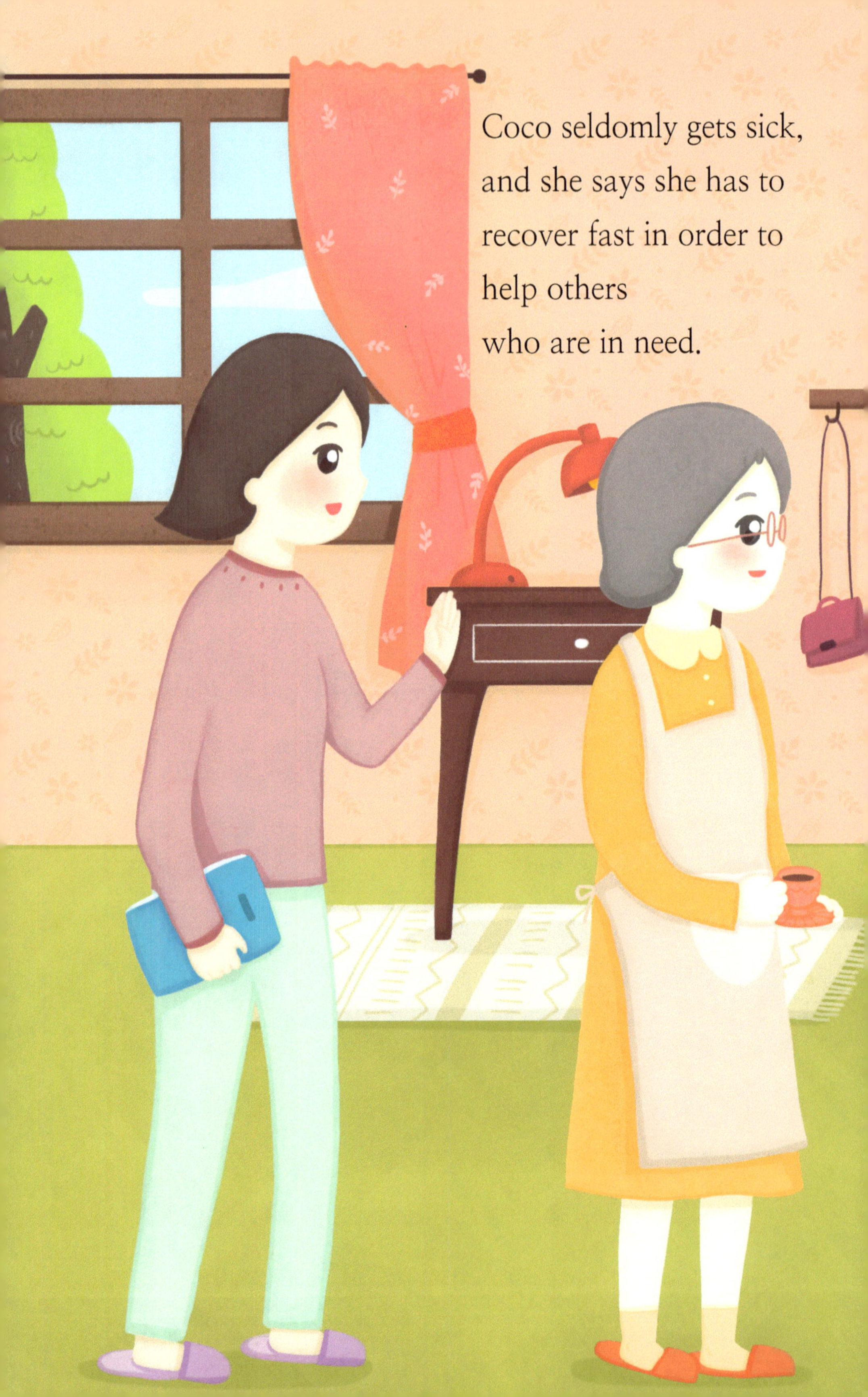

Coco seldomly gets sick,
and she says she has to
recover fast in order to
help others
who are in need.

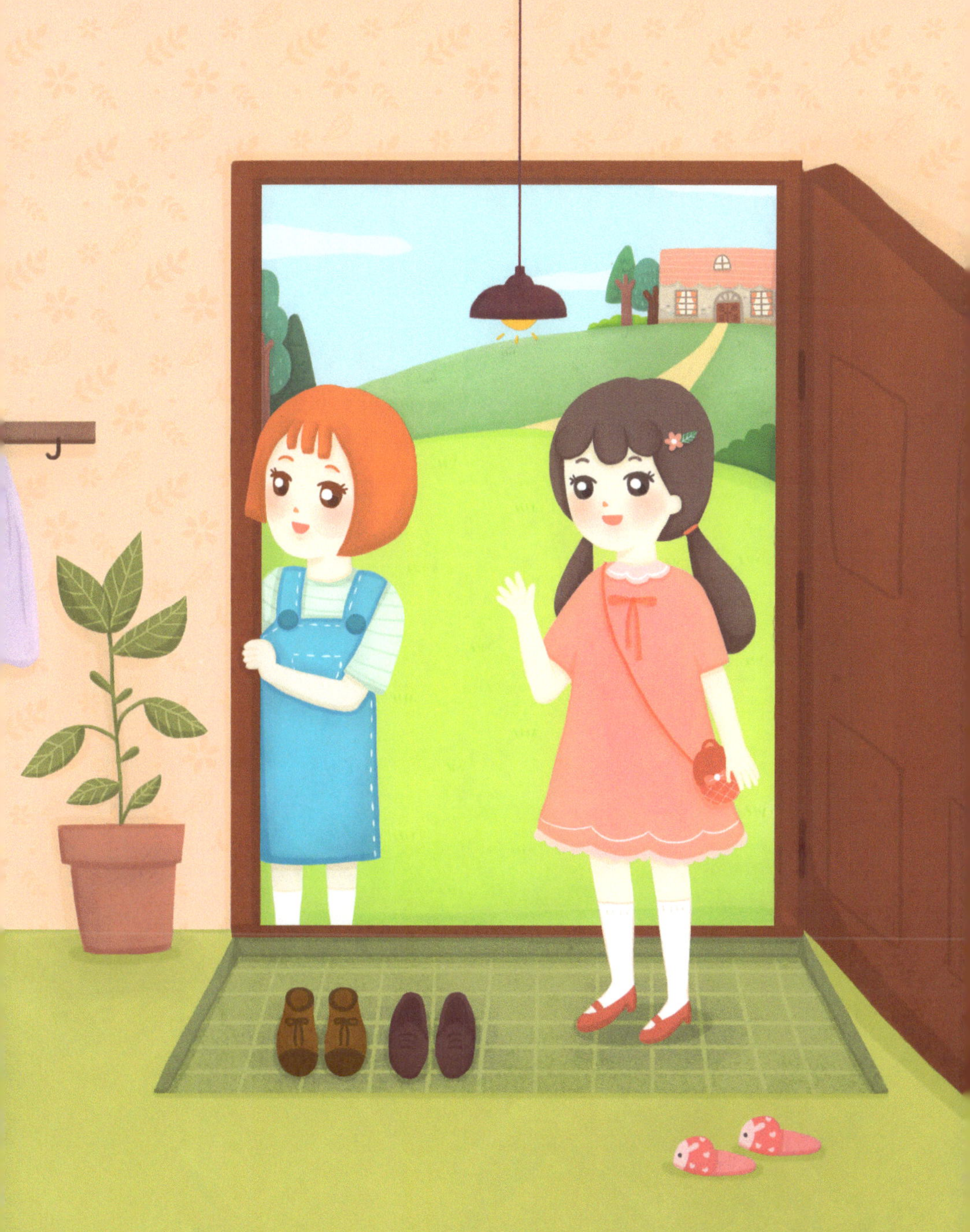

She gets recovered from the help
of her mother and grandmother.

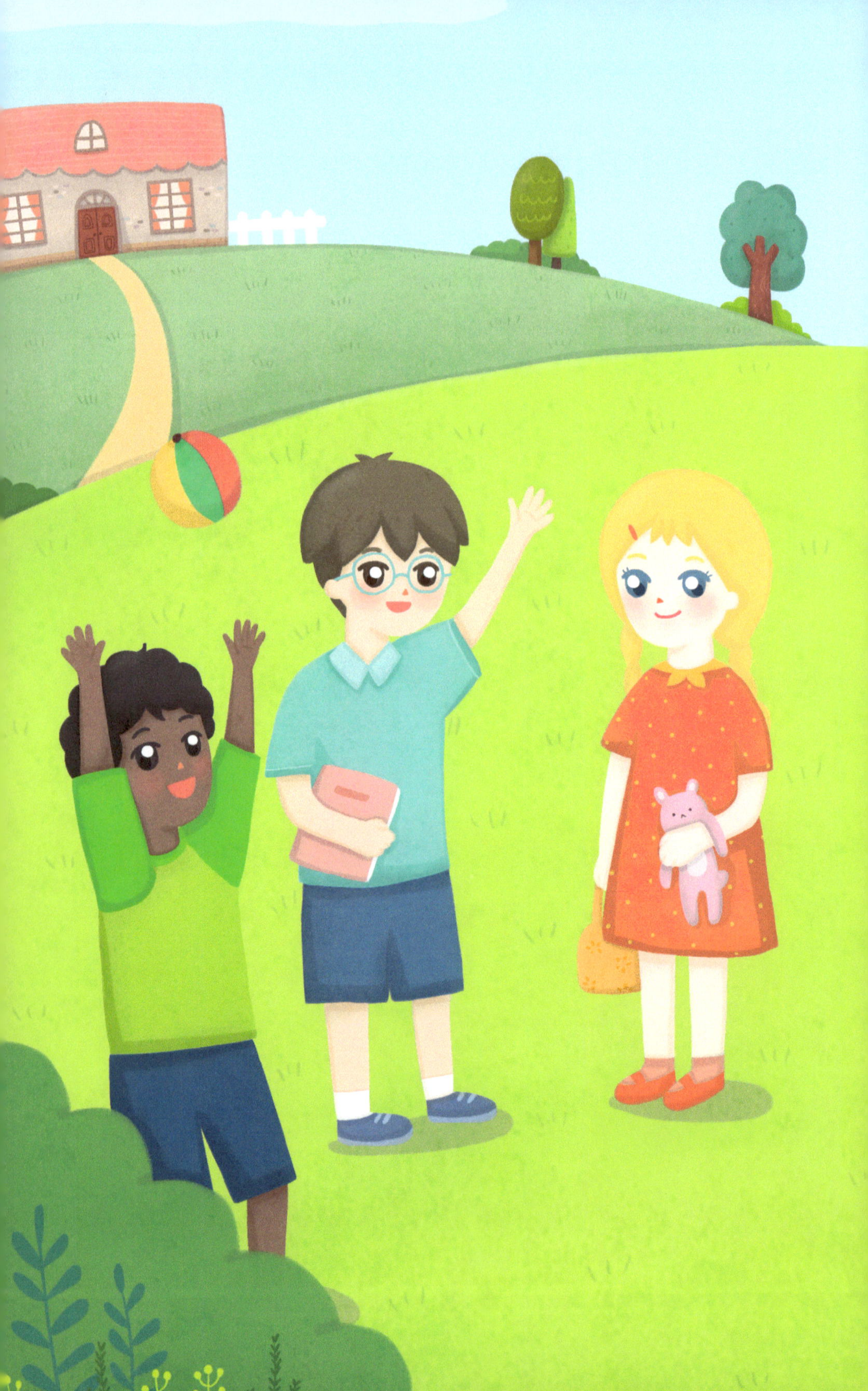

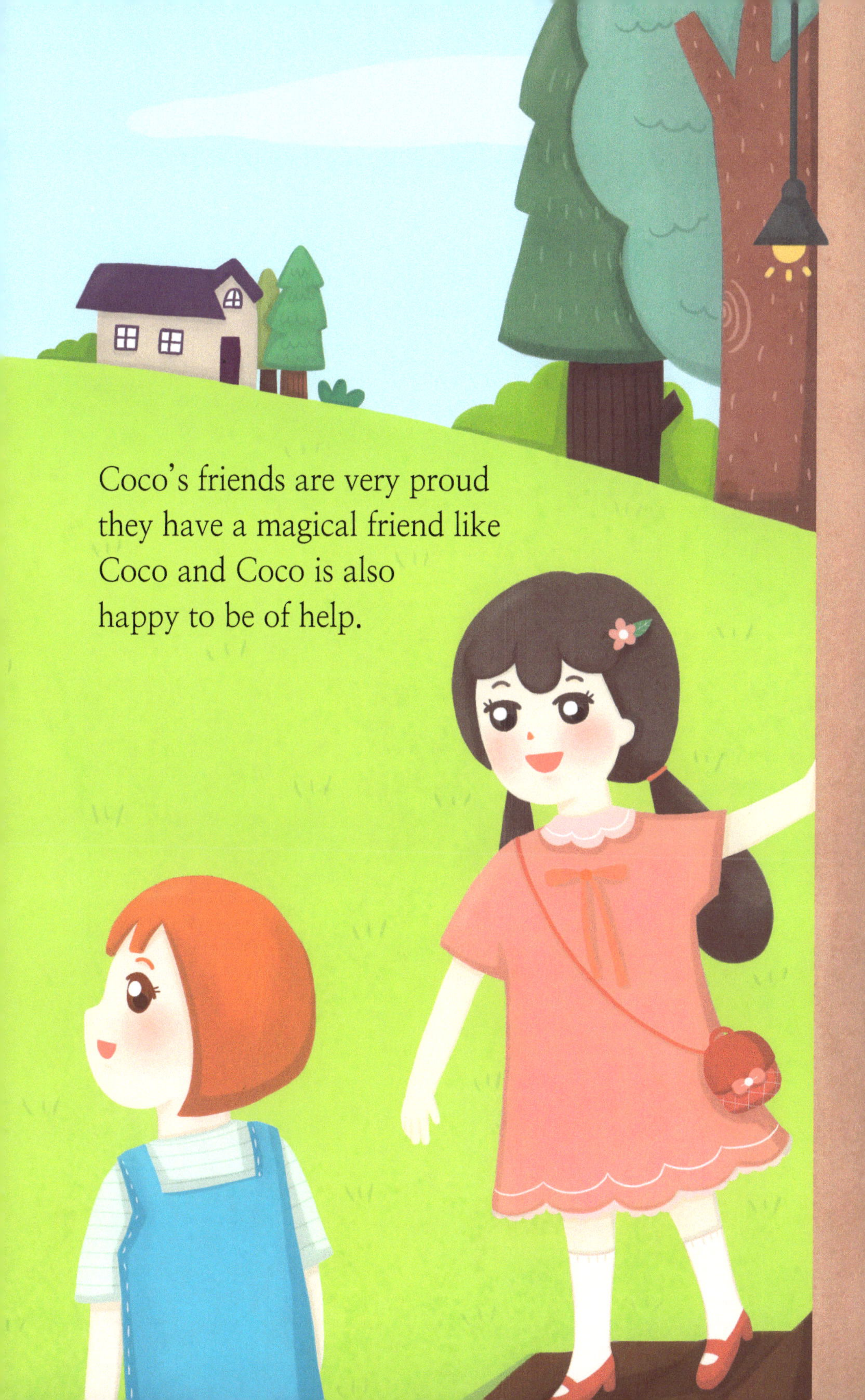

Coco's friends are very proud
they have a magical friend like
Coco and Coco is also
happy to be of help.

What is herbal medicine?

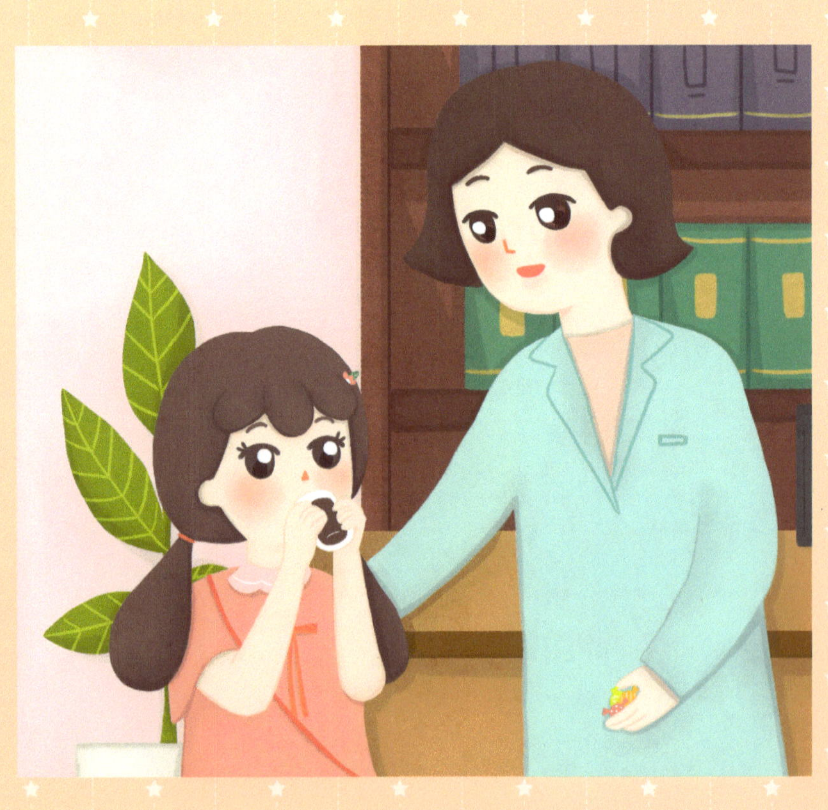

What is herbal medicine?

Herbal medicine is a mixture of herbs from nature.

Like other medicines, it makes us healthy.

The most common form is liquid form.

Some tastes sour or bitter, but it is okay after

a while. Sometimes I only have to take one day's

amount, while there are times I have to take the

herbal medicine for more than a month.

I like herbal medicine because it makes me stay

healthy. It also makes me feel happy.

Author

Jeongmin Ko K.M.D. and Hyojung Kwon K.M.D.

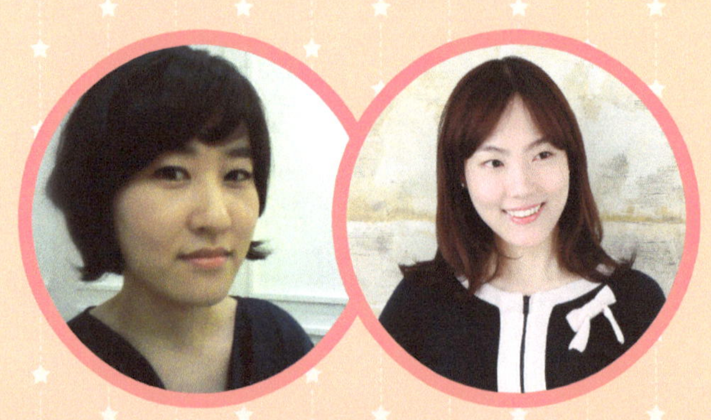

Graduates of School of Korean medicine, Kyunghee University and trained in the department of acupuncture and moxibustion, Kyunghee University hospital, the two authors currently practice Korean medicine in Bundang and Daegu, Korea. The authors want to show the world the wonders of Korean medicine.

Illustrator
Ji Eun Jeon

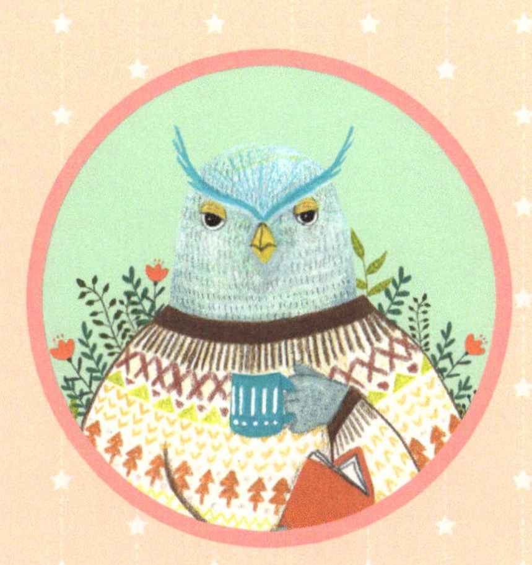

Hello, I am Ji Eun Jeon, an illustrator who draws pictures of everyday life. I wish my pictures can help people share ideas. It was a fascinating project for me to meet 'Coco', a magical girl, and illustrate her story in the summer of 2016. I hope the story of Coco's family and friends bring Korean medicine one step closer to everyone.